PLAYING GAMES –

LOSING WEIGHT –

LIVING LIFE –

By Peg Grossi

ISBN: 1-4033-7791-X (Electronic)
ISBN: 1-4033-7792-8 (Softcover)

This book is printed on acid free paper.

1stBooks – rev. 09/12/02

The advice and exercises presented in this book are in no way intended as a substitute for medical counseling.

Consult your doctor before beginning this or any other diet program.

The author, publisher, and distributors of Playing Games – Losing Weight – Living Life – disclaim any liability or loss in connection with the advise herein.

Dedicated to my children and grandchildren who, because of their own accomplishments, inspired me to write this book.

It is also in memory of my beloved husband whose guidance and influence throughout all of our lives made us what we are today – successful in our happiness.

Thank you Peter. We love you.

TABLE OF CONTENTS

PLAYING GAMES —

LOSING WEIGHT –

LIVING LIFE –

You have tried every diet in every dieting book ever published which have been written by dietitians, nutritionists, weight counselors, Hollywood celebrities — even doctors. Right? Of course, right!

There was the Atkins Diet – The Suzanne Somers Diet – The Cabbage Soup Diet — The Jenny Craig Program — Weight Watchers — The Lazy Lady's Diet — The New Guide to Intelligent Reducing Diet – The 9-Day Wonder Diet – The Mayo Clinic Diet – The Woman Doctor's Diet – The Pritikin Program – The LaCosta Diet – The One Meal A Day Diet – The All Vegetable Diet – The All Protein Diet.

Have I hit upon any one of your diets yet? Probably not, because there are more of them out there for your perusal than you could possibly shake a chicken drumstick at.

You've heard about them from real friends who are 100 per cent behind your weight loss efforts. You've heard about them from your enemies who don't want you to be successful at losing weight (I hope you don't have too many of those.) You've read about them in beauty magazines featuring pencil-thin, glamorous models, in thick verbose books, and in newspapers. You've seen them extolled in television commercials, on the internet, and even on roadside billboards. You've listened to them being pitched over radio airwaves — to the point where you've become nauseated.

You've gone over and over a myriad of diets in your mind and, quite often, have even tried them for a week or two. You <u>really</u> did try to make them work. BUT you just couldn't tolerate the monotony of the foods — or the lack of same.

You must have noticed by now that I haven't even mentioned the multitudinous DIETING AIDS that are on the market today – those chemical products that promise to take innumerable pounds off by simply ingesting them. I refuse to give them even a modicum of space in this book because they're not worthy of any intelligent coverage whatsoever. They have been proven to be unequivocally ineffectual and, quite often, harmful to your health. Suffice it to say, no one at all should succumb to the persistent hype about them. They're strictly a waste of my time, your time, and your money.

Let's face it. <u>Almost </u>any diet you try will work for a short period of time — during the time that you stick to it. Note the fact that I said <u>almost</u>. Most of them don't work at all, but even though in your heart you suspect that they don't, you're still willing to give them a try. So you try. You stick to it for a few weeks and, if you're lucky, you lose a few pounds. However, when you return to your usual eating habits, those few pounds inevitably return with a vengeance. To add insult to injury, you have most likely even gained a few more. Undoubtedly you dropped the diet and felt frustrated enough to go on an eating binge. Who could blame you?

I'm positive you will become inspired by simply reading about this plan which enables you to lose weight as well as being a health program, but just being inspired is not sufficient enough to lose weight. You realize this because you've gone through this many, many times before.

You need something more powerful. Think about it. You need to be MOTIVATED each and every day to follow any program to its fruition to be able to reap results.

This program will enable you to easily accomplish this. IT WILL KEEP YOU MOTIVATED. IT WILL KEEP YOU ON TRACK. IT WILL KEEP YOU INSPIRED. The numerous CRUTCHES and dieting aids (not chemical) of this program will keep you interested because you, alone, have the option to choose a different crutch each day. You, alone, will decide how you want to play the game to lose your weight.

The way you utilize this program is determined by YOU. YOU MAKE THE RULES. YOU are in charge of the formula each and every day of your life. I say for your life because once you've gotten into this program you'll never want to live without it again.

Whichever crutch you choose is the one YOU want to implement that day. No one else is making your choice for you, or setting any specific rules. YOU keep it interesting by selecting whatever crutch is interesting to YOU. YOU decide how much of yourself you're going to put into the program that particular day — or even if you're going to skip that day. Yes, you do have the option of skipping a day or two which, as you have learned, is almost never permitted in any other diet plan.

AND IT'S ABSOLUTELY FREE!! YES, I SAID FREE!! There are absolutely, positively, unconditionally no membership dues to pay each and every week (regardless of whether or not you lost any weight that week.)

Even taking for granted that you own a video cassette recorder, there are no video tapes to invest in. Video tapes are only beneficial if you use them daily. When you neglect to use them for a few days they eventually end up gathering dust on your shelves.

The same is true for any diet audio tapes that might be in existence. They would not be as interesting as the video tapes and would be much easier to ignore. They would be much easier to banish to your bottom drawer which houses all of the other items you never use.

Another great advantage to this program is that there are no special meals to purchase, which other diet programs require you to do. These meals could be duplicated in your own home at a fraction of the cost and would, most likely, taste even better. There is still another great advantage. There are no gym fees to pay.

No contracts to sign. No sweat suits or workout outfits to buy. No glamorous, thin bodies to compete with. NO INVESTMENT WHATSOEVER

Just as you did, I tried an endless number of diets and after many years of yo-yo dieting I came to the undeniable conclusion that the only absolutely certain way to lose weight — permanently — is to change HOW you eat, not WHAT you eat.

Everyone knows you <u>will</u> lose some weight providing you entirely eliminate breads, cheeses, bacon, pastas with heavy sauces, all desserts, and trim ALL fat from meats. In other words, you give up almost everything which is pleasing to the palate.

If you are blessed with a tremendous amount of will power and discipline you may be able to stay on that diet for a short period of time.

BUT, REALISTICALLY, HOW LONG CAN YOU DEPRIVE YOURSELF OF THE INHERENT PLEASURE OF EATING THE FOOD YOU ENJOY THE MOST? After a few weeks (or for even that long) of constantly salivating and chewing your nails to the nub while watching other people devour their <u>rich,</u> fat-laden entrees or <u>rich,</u> luscious desserts (of course, chocolate is your supreme favorite flavor), you come to the inevitable following conclusion: <u>Nothing</u>, not even a svelte, hard, trim body like your favorite movie celebrity's or your favorite rock star's is worth such a horrendous, humungous sacrifice.

YOU DECIDE TO GIVE INTO TEMPTATION and consume your heart's (and stomach's) desire. You have extraordinarily little trouble convincing yourself that "it's only this one time". Ah, but there's the rub. It isn't only this one time. You've deprived yourself of your cravings for too long a time. YOU GO OFF YOUR DIET! You return to eating the way you did prior to this latest attempt at dieting and losing weight. How many old college tries have you given it? How many times has it been? Ten? Twenty? More?

BUT TAKE HEART! Here is your answer, your key, your solution, your salvation. This is the program you've been seeking all of your adult life. Perhaps your parents were looking for it for you as a child.

Now, here is the program you'll be telling your friends about when they ask you how you've lost all your excess weight. You won't be able to resist talking about it even if they don't ask you to. You'll be so overflowing with enthusiasm, you'll want to climb on rooftops to exclaim what's happened to you. Well, maybe not. I'm sure though that you will be happy for having tried it.

Here is the program (I will not diminish its effectiveness by calling it a diet) to end all other diets. IT WORKS. It works because YOU make it work. You're in complete control. You make it what you want it to be. YOU make it fun. YOU make it interesting.

IT WORKS.

As I told you before, I've been there.

Take it from someone who has been on most of the usual diets, as you were, and then after losing a few pounds was not able to keep them off. Take it from someone who finally became desperate enough to devise this program. Take it from someone who has been there and is living proof that IT WORKS. I have been using these dieting aids (CRUTCHES) for several years now. Let me tell you that my weight fluctuates only 1 & 3 lbs. monthly.

THE FORMULA

Unless I've missed my guess, I'm reasonably certain that by now I've sufficiently whetted your interest to the point where you want to find out just what this wonder program consists of.

You wouldn't be seeking out books about how to lose weight if you weren't hoping to find yet another diet that will help you lose a few pounds to help achieve that ideal body you've always yearned for. You're cognizant of the fact that you've tried numerous diets with very few results (or none at all). Nevertheless you know you just can't help yourself. You need to give it another try. You hope that MAYBE, JUST MAYBE, this one will work. Well, you're in luck. You are now reading the last book you will ever have to read on the subject.

Are you ready for this? HERE'S THE SECRET FORMULA.

"PLAYING GAMES – LOSING WEIGHT – LIVING LIFE –" is based on the same concept as one, I would imagine, almost everyone has heard about at one time or another. It is the Alcoholics Anonymous program which advocates facing a drinking problem ONE DAY AT A TIME. This program tackles losing weight ONE DAY AT A TIME. Honestly, it's that simple.

You choose one CRUTCH each and every day and during the time you're fulfilling that crutch you console yourself that <u>is</u> FOR ONE DAY ONLY and that "tomorrow – if I want to – I'll be able to go back to my old ways and indulge in that particular goody again".

If you are a Christian you have, most likely, made sacrifices during the Lenten period. You were taught to do so as a child. Perhaps you are still engaging in this practice as an adult. It's a habit ingrained in you — an excellent one.

In all likelihood, you have given up eating between meals, smoking, or drinking, promised to exercise, or attend service in your church daily.

Undoubtedly you were successful in doing so because your pledge to abstain was going to be for only the length of the Lenten season. You could hardly wait for Easter Sunday because you knew you could, again, have whatever food or activity of which you deprived yourself. You were able to achieve your specific goal because each and every time you found yourself weakening you assuaged your craving by reinforcing the fact that your sacrifice was for a limited length of time only.

From my own experience, during the time that I was a smoker (29 years ago) I would always vow to smoke only one cigarette an hour for the length of the Lenten season.

Keep in mind that I consumed two packages of cigarettes daily. I was able to keep my promise because I knew it was for a limited period of time. I must confess, though, that I always stayed up past the midnight hour just to indulge myself in the last cigarette for the day.

Having been smoke-free for the last 29 years I now realize what a weak person I was – and am. I need structure in my life. That's why I devised this program. I need it.

Psych yourself up daily. Upon waking in the morning, think about how you're going to definitely lose some weight today. This day. Picture how you will look in your new clothes with your new figure and also reflect upon how much more energy you'll going to have. Ponder carefully about how improving yourself today will benefit you long term.

Every time you use a particular crutch, psych yourself up by saying to yourself "right at this moment I am losing a few ounces or even a pound that will be added to my ultimate accumulative weight loss." The motivation you feel and the sense of accomplishment you derive immediately far outweighs the effort you need to expel. The high you get is truly euphoric. Who needs drugs?

To be able to achieve the euphoria I'm talking about, you need only to learn and execute this simple program. What do you have to lose? Absolutely nothing except some weight. On the other hand, you gain immensely in the way of health and happiness.

Ready to try? Great! Let's go.

<u>YOUR 49 CRUTCHES</u>

1. SEEK HELP

We all know that the most difficult part of any endeavor is disciplining yourself to follow through. It's impossible to do this alone — by yourself. There is a huge gap between motivation and implementation. The most important thing you need to do is to fill that gap.

Again, take heart. There is the ultimate crutch available to you – one that you could have thought of yourself if you had just taken some time for concentration and a little meditation whenever you experienced any kind of predicament. You could have used it each time you tackled any one of your previous diets. What is necessary to do is to elicit help from the Powers That Be — your God, Lord, Jehovah, Allah, Yaweh, Buddha, Isis, Wolan, Zeus, or from whatever source you derive help during your daily life. You promise Him or Her that, for this ONE DAY you will eliminate the particular food you chose, or you will perform one of the dieting aids which you will learn about shortly.

2. PROMISE YOUR SUPREME BEING that you will stick to the program for at least one week. It is at this point in the program – at the beginning – that you need His help the most. The initial attempt is the most difficult. The first week is fraught with pitfalls because you won't be accustomed to ignoring any of the foods which you have not chosen as a crutch.

Remember that the program is for ONE DAY AT A TIME and you will be able to get through your first week easier than you thought you could. Pardon the pun, but it'll be as easy as duck's soup.

Choose a crutch that doesn't normally appeal to you. If you love chocolate, don't give it up for one day. Give up something instead that doesn't entice your taste buds.

You may not notice a reduction in your weight consistently each day but I personally guarantee that if you persist for at least a week there <u>will</u> be a change in your weight. You won't even have an opportunity to use an eighth of the crutches available to you.

3. WHEN TO CHOOSE YOUR
CRUTCH FOR THE DAY

Choose your daily aid (or crutch) at the same time each day. How about the first thing upon arising? You could set your alarm for five minutes earlier than necessary and just lie there and make your choice for the day. After a remarkably short time you will know all of the crutches by heart. If you have ever taken a few minutes to relax completely before getting out of bed, you know what a wonderful feeling it can be. What a great time to both relax and also get your motivation for the day!

You could also use the relaxing time in the shower to make your selection. You could do it while brushing your teeth. You could use your daily exercise sessions (which is really an excellent time to combine the two actions which will lead to weight loss). We will delve into specific exercises later on in this book.

The point I'm trying to make here is that choosing your crutch the first thing in the morning, every morning at the same time while performing the same hygienic regimen, leads into it becoming a habit — you know, like brushing your teeth, taking a shower, or exercising. You just don't think twice about doing them. They're habits. They're a part of your life. So, choosing your crutch will also become the best habit you will ever cultivate.

This step is paramount to the success of this program. It is only next of importance to your making the commitment in the first place.

Once you get into the habit of choosing your crutch for the day you're off and running.

The best part of choosing your crutch is that you don't need to isolate your mind to make the choice. You don't need to concentrate on it singularly. You can be doing something else at the same time. Hence, also performing the hygiene habits mentioned above.

You can also include your choice during your morning prayer time. What better time than while talking to your Supreme Being? You asked Him to help you in your decision to start, didn't you?

4. WEIGH YOURSELF
   EACH AND EVERY DAY

Oh, I know there are doctors, nutritionists, weight trainers, personal counselors, and various diet experts who would disagree with me vehemently regarding this unprecedented theory. There is a method to my madness. In order for this program to be effective, you must know how much you weigh each day. How else will you know if it is, indeed, working?

As I said before, this program works <u>one day at a time.</u> After the first day of using one of the crutches, if you lose a pound, or even if only a half-pound, the euphoria you will experience will give you the incentive to continue......to go on tomorrow. If you don't weigh in at any less, you'll rationalize that whatever particular food you eliminated for the day wasn't the most efficient to constitute a loss of weight. You tell yourself that you'll be more successful tomorrow.

You can see that either way, on this program it's imperative to weigh yourself every day — and also at the same time of day. It's psychologically prudent to do so.

I weigh myself each day the first thing upon arising — before I place anything at all into my stomach. (After all, that cup of coffee <u>may weigh an ounce or so.)</u> Then I record my weight in that day's block on a calendar. The next morning I compare to see whether I've lost or gained. This is where the techniques in the above paragraph come into play.

At the end of each month I average the numbers and compare them to the previous month. I'm extremely satisfied when the numbers remain the same and am not too concerned if there is a fluctuation of a pound one way or the other. I use the same procedure at the end of the year.

As I told you, this is a game I've been playing for years. It's a game that reminds me constantly to continue working at keeping myself healthy and trim. It's also a game I enjoy thoroughly.

5. DRINK 8 GLASSES
OF WATER DAILY

To hasten the process, you must drink at least 8 glasses of water daily. Here is where all the other diet hucksters and I agree. I know that I'm being redundant but this step is <u>extremely important.</u> Not only will you lose the weight more quickly, you'll be cleansing your entire system each and every day, creating better health and a smoother, lovelier complexion.

This step is really easy to carry out.

Fill a pitcher with 64 ounces of this miracle beverage. Fill a glass and then refill it every time it gets low. Carry it with you into every room — wherever you go. Keep sipping it whenever your glance falls on it while you're doing your chores. Before you know it you will have drunk all 64 ounces — ONE SIP AT A TIME! May your cup runneth over. (I couldn't resist that one).

If you don't want a pitcher cluttering up your counter all day, you can keep an 8-ounce glass filled constantly at arm's reach, (keeping count of how many times you filled it.) Of course, you <u>could</u> drink more than 64 ounces if you'd like to. You'll find yourself sipping more frequently than is needed, and you won't even realize that you've reached your goal.

Don't worry about having to live in the ladies' (or men's) room because of this extra water consumption. Your bladder will compensate after a few days and your system will become cleansed with no effort at all.

Oh yes, by the way, you cannot substitute coffee, tea, soda, orange, grapefruit, prune, guava, or <u>any other kind of juices or liquids</u> for your glass of water.

I like a slice of lemon in my water but when I don't have any lemons in the refrigerator I simply use a little bottled lemon juice. In the summer I add a few ice cubes. In the winter I add hot water. I'm fortunate to have a boiling water dispenser in my kitchen sink so it's a breeze to make the hot lemonade. Hey, you might not like lemon in your water – so drink it plain. Whatever works for you.

Three of those glasses of water should be consumed just prior to eating your breakfast, lunch, and dinner. Not only will this make a big dent in the 64 ounces you need to drink daily, but you'll be amazed at how only one glass of water before eating will curb your appetite for each meal.

I can actually feel your annoyance as you're reading this saying, "sure <u>you</u> can do this — you most likely stay at home all day, but <u>I work for a living</u>". Well, you're only partially correct. I work part-time and if I haven't consumed my eight glasses of water before I leave for work at 2:00 P.M., I take a water bottle with me (you know, one of those sports bottles that are all the rage these days).

If you don't happen to have a water supply at your workplace, join the water bottle crowd and you're in like Flynn. There is absolutely no reason in the world why you can't finish off that 64 ounces of water each and every day. It's a necessary element to maintain your system in tip-top running condition and it's simple to do.

6. KEEP YOUR SYSTEM REGULAR

Because this program allows you to eat every conceivable food in existence, it is an extremely healthy way to lose weight. Every vitamin or mineral known to man is consumed at one time or another.

There is one important thing I do religiously, however, no matter which crutch I choose for the day, and that's to be certain that my system remains regular at all times. To accomplish this I make certain to have a small amount of cereal daily. Sometimes it's bran, sometimes wheat, sometimes a combination. I also have one or two prunes which are either raw or stewed. I can't remember the last time I had to take a chemical laxative.

I eat the cereal just before retiring in the evening. Allowing myself to eat the cereal has a psychological benefit over and above the physical benefit also. There are days when I've deprived myself of one of my favorite foods for the day, and I look forward to eating "my laxative." My rules, you know.

7. EAT ONLY HALF PORTIONS

In the event that you possess a ravenous appetite, eating only half portions may be the <u>only </u>dieting crutch you will need. Nevertheless, you really should try some of the other crutches because you'll experience the FUN of playing the dieting game and you'll definitely be able to lose even more weight.

If you have chosen giving up snacks for the day, measure out only half of the amount you would usually eat each time you reach for one.

Before each meal serve yourself only half of the amount again, consuming only half the amount of calories. You'll be surprised at how satisfied you'll be without gorging yourself. If you choose this crutch for several days in a row, eating smaller portions may very well become a habit. By disciplining yourself to eat only half portions at every meal you will also be gradually shrinking your stomach.

Eventually you will actually be <u>unable</u> to consume as much as you formerly did

This is an especially beneficial crutch to use during the Thanksgiving and Christmas feeding frenzies. It's almost impossible (unless you're an extremely strong-willed person) to give up any one type of food during these holidays, but you can certainly make a promise to eat only half the amounts you would normally devour. You won't be deprived of any of the seasonal goodies.

Think of the parties you'll be attending where you won't be able to avoid the delicious repasts on all of the buffet tables or the irresistible hors d'oeuvre being served non-stop. And, be honest, you really don't want to!! But you <u>can</u> limit your intake of these diet busters.

Then there are those numerous invitations for those sumptuous luncheons and dinners which make November and December virtual dieting pitfall months.

All of these food snares can at least be partially avoided if you tackle them with your resolve to eat only half of what you did during last year's holiday season.

8. EAT VERY SLOWLY

This is an extremely easy crutch to use. Today you don't have to limit your intake. You just have to take at least 15 minutes to eat every meal. It has been proven that if you eat slowly your appetite is satisfied more quickly. Consequently, you consume fewer calories every time you put something into your mouth.

If you've been accustomed to inhaling your food, it may be difficult to slow yourself down. When you begin to eat, you're going to have to remind yourself of what you are trying to accomplish. Think of the weight you're going to lose. You'll slow down considerably if you picture yourself in that new outfit you tried on last week which didn't fit.

While you're eating slowly you'll be amazed at how tasty the food is. You'll savor every bite, appreciate and enjoy the fragrances, flavors, and textures. Eating will become a pleasurable experience instead of only something to do to keep yourself healthy.

9. CHEW EACH PIECE OF FOOD THOROUGHLY

This crutch goes hand-in-hand with the previous one (Eat Very Slowly) and the one that follows (Leave a Little Bit of Food on Your Plate). If you choose one of them for the day you'll probably find yourself performing the others also.

Medical research has proven that chewing each piece of food at least 8 times before swallowing helps to digest it better. Digesting your food better also makes for a healthier digestive system. A healthier digestive system makes a healthier person. How much simpler can this concept be?

In addition, chewing thoroughly may even prevent a person from having a choking incident. Eating too fast is the primary cause of choking.

Chewing thoroughly, eating slowly, or using any other crutch will remind you of <u>why</u> you are changing your eating habits. It's to LOSE WEIGHT.

10. LEAVE A LITTLE BIT OF FOOD ON YOUR PLATE

There is a television ad for a diet product that starts with "if you could leave a little bit of food on your plate at every meal, think of how much weight you could lose in a month" (or something to that effect). And it's true.

It works on the same principle as limiting yourself to half-portions – except that it does not work as quickly. It will probably only allow you to cut 100 calories for the day but those 100 calories a day will add up in the long run if, after choosing this crutch for a few days, it becomes a consistent habit.— There's that definitive word again. Habit.

As I said earlier on, it's not WHAT you eat – it's HOW you eat. If you can teach yourself to eat slowly, eat less, leave food on your plate at each meal and make it a HABIT to live with, you'll never have to worry about maintaining your weight loss.

Trust me. It works.

11. DON'T SAMPLE WHILE COOKING

Today you're expecting guests for dinner and you're going to be cooking and baking for most of the day. It's a perfect day to promise to use this crutch. You're going to be tempted to taste the ingredients of the appetizers, the entrée, the vegetables, the salad, the rolls, and the dessert. You tell yourself that it's imperative that you sample the ingredients to make certain that the meal will be perfect.

Not so. You <u>may</u> need to taste once or twice but, come on now – be truthful, how often do you pick at an ingredient, or lick a spoon, or scrape a pan, when it isn't really necessary? I'll venture to say it's a lot more often than you care to admit.

Now, think of the hundreds of calories you'll consume just <u>preparing</u> the meal, even before you start eating it with your guests. Get into the HABIT of not sampling the food while cooking your family's daily meals also.

Isn't it coincidental that many chefs border on the obese? True, there are many who do not, but perhaps they are the ones who, without exception, do not sample while cooking. They have never succumbed to this objectionable habit.

This particular crutch is especially beneficial to chefs or their apprentices, for those who do not have the self-discipline to refrain from tasting their creations every step of the way, ignoring the fact that they are adding to their caloric intake. They certainly know this is the price they have to pay but they need to have a crutch — they need this program.

You have the advantage of reading this book and gaining the knowledge you need. You will become more aware of where the pitfalls are hidden. It isn't that you were not cognizant of them before you picked up this book. Now, however, you will learn how to contend with them — how to fight the temptations they put forth.

12. COOK AN ENTIRELY DIETETIC MEAL

If you enjoy cooking at all, this will be an intriguing challenge. A person who enjoys playing chef enjoys every phase of it — shopping for the ingredients, measuring out the amounts of each one, mixing, blending, cooking or baking. Every step is a joy to execute.

And this is just when you prepare your regular recipes. Imagine how exciting it would be to have a brand new – exciting — cooking experience!

You can borrow numerous dietetic books from your local library. In addition, the trip to the library will be rewarding for you. You will also be able to add to your own library of regular recipes plus the dietetic ones. These books contain recipes from soup to nuts. Complete meals. You'll have a ball cooking this "almost no caloric meal" Again, refrain from munching on the ingredients while preparing it.

13.   UTILIZE PREPARED
DIETETIC MEALS

So you're not Julia Child or Jacques Pepin. You don't know a spatula from a cleaver. And what's more, you don't care. You <u>don't like to cook.</u> You would love to take control of your low fat, low caloric intake but you just don't have the skills to cook up a healthy, dietetic meal.

Take heart.   There are so many already prepared dietetic meals on the market that you could have one for breakfast, one for lunch and still another one for dinner.   Granted, you <u>would</u> lose weight if you ate nothing but those kind of meals.   However, regardless of what they feature, these commercially prepared foods eventually take on pretty much the same tastes and flavor. The answer here is to us any one of these products for ONE DAY ONLY — occasionally — and you will lose a half pound or so to add to your cumulative weight loss. It's just another crutch for you to play the game with. Remember, IT'S A GAME.

14. POSTPONE DESSERT

When you have just completed a meal during which you either ate slowly, or had only half portions, or only ate everything which was completely dietetic, or have left something on your plate, you will, most likely, want to reward yourself by finishing it off with a scrumptious, mouth-watering dessert.

Make postponing dessert your crutch for the day. You will not have it immediately following the meal. Clear the table, load the dishwasher, and hand wash the pots and pans. This can also be the perfect opportunity to train your family to help you clean up before any of you indulge in dessert. It'll become a habit— one of the many good habits you'll acquire during this program.

After I clean up I may decide that I don't want any dessert at all, but if I do indulge myself, it will be with a considerably smaller portion than it would have been had I not given myself time to think about the extra calories I would consume. I remember that it's just for today. I may think differently tomorrow.

15. ELIMINATE DESSERT
ENTIRELY

Here's a revolutionary thought!! For today, and because it <u>is</u> only for the one day, you will give up anything that even resembles dessert. You may rationalize that peanut butter and jelly on a cracker is more in the cracker category — but it's still dessert. And don't forget those dangerous between meal sweets – candy, cup cakes, brownies. You know them all.

There are many categories of foods that might fit into both the entrée category or the dessert category (jello for instance), but don't let them fool you. THEY REALLY ARE DESSERTS. If you are honest with yourself you'll end up losing at least a pound or two.

This crutch may even be easier for you than postponing dessert or having a half-portion of same. Sometimes just the smallest taste of a forbidden food is enough to trigger the desire for a larger portion. Sometime it's better — and easier — to abstain entirely.

16. BANISH CHOCOLATE FOR TODAY

Yes, chocolate. You may be thinking that you don't even like chocolates all that much. You're talking about chocolate candy. It's almost inconceivable how chocolate finds its way into a myriad of other foods and, subsequently, finds its way into your unsuspecting stomach — and fat cells.

Take breakfast for instance. You don't normally think of chocolate as a breakfast food, but there are some people who like hot chocolate instead of coffee at that time of day. Then there are the chocolate chip pancakes or waffles. How about the cereals which contain chocolate, such as cocoa puffs? Then there are the irresistible chocolate spreads for your toast, rolls, or muffins.

Lunch and dinner present even more of a problem. There are so many main entrees that contain chocolate and no one could ever list the chocolate desserts in existence. Chocolate between-meal snacks also run rampant. Chocolate rules!

17. ELIMINATE BETWEEN MEAL SNACKS

This is an extremely effective crutch in order to shed a few pounds, especially if you're notorious for munching between meals. I don't happen to be a muncher so I don't use it very often but I may if I want to stay the course of the program. (I told you that everyone on this program makes up their own rules.)

However, if you do have that vice, this crutch will be very advantageous in helping you to lose weight quickly. If you keep your promise and also use it for several times a week, you'll see results very soon.

It won't be easy to check yourself each time you see your hand reaching for a cookie, a cracker, an apple, an orange, or <u>anything at all.</u> Sipping some of your required 64-ounces of water will help. Even if you've already consumed the 64 ounces you'll be able to substitute the water for the snack. Now you have polished off two of the crutches and reinforced your resolve to stick to the program ONE DAY AT A TIME!

18. PASS UP ALL BREADS AND/OR ROLLS

It has been statistically proven that by simply eliminating all breads and rolls from your diet you can shed a significant amount of weight – in a very short time. If you're like me though, that would be like asking you to give up breathing.

I LOVE rye bread, white bread, wheat bread, garlic bread, rosemary with oil bread, raisin bread, et cetera, et cetera, et cetera.

I also LOVE every type of roll known to man, including all muffins, from English to corn. And, of course, I can't eat them without the fattening, fattening butter. More calories!

I can lose up to a couple of pounds if I use this crutch for just two days. If you don't consistently devour breads and rolls on a daily basis like I do, don't waste your time using this crutch. You could, however, use it if you want an easy day in order to stay on the program and to keep playing the losing game. Anything to keep yourself focused on your ultimate goal – weight loss.

19. EXCLUDE MARGARINE

You would think that passing up the breads and rolls is enough to keep you safe from this particular peril. Not so.

I would venture to say that you have never been aware of how many times a day you eat butter or margarine, or how many ways you use it in cooking. Besides as a spread, there are a myriad of recipes which contain it... from a teaspoonful to a cup or more. TALK ABOUT EXTRA CALORIES!

If you can possibly exclude it once in a while for one day — use it for your crutch — your total calories for the day will be cut considerably.   Of course you wouldn't eliminate it for an extended period of time. That would make life extremely tasteless.

But you <u>could</u> attempt to use it at least for one day.

Each day that you choose a crutch and make your promise to your Supreme Being becomes a new experience. It's a new game— each and every day.

20. GIVE UP ALL CHEESES

There are so many tempting cheeses available today — American, Blue, Brie, Cheddar, Cottage, Cream, Muenster, Swiss – more than I could possibly name here. And they're all delicious. I don't know anyone who doesn't like cheese. If a diet forces them to limit their intake, they find ways to get low fat or fat free. It may not taste as good as the genuine, but at least some of the taste is there.

Cheese is a food we consume in so very many ways, whether eating it alone or utilizing it in endless ways to make appetizers, main courses, or desserts. It's even universally popular in omelets for breakfast.

It's another food that I couldn't live without. You're most likely thinking that almost every food is my favorite— and you're right. I TOLD YOU, I LOVE TO EAT.

That's why I find this program so easy to follow. I CAN give up my favorite food for one day at a time, knowing that I can have it again the next day if I so desire.

21. HAVE A SALAD DAY

This is my daughter's favorite crutch because she would rather eat salads than any other kind of food. I, personally, don't care very much for them so I don't use this crutch very often. However, I do use it when I want to lose some weight quickly.

Remember though, you can't freely drench any kind of salad with fatty dressings. That would just defeat the purpose. There are a great variety of fat-free dressings on the market if you don't want to take the trouble of making your own vinaigrette.

You can, of course, stretch the SALAD crutch a bit. Do you realize how many different foods can justifiably fit into the salad category? There's egg salad, tuna salad, chicken salad, crab meat salad, et cetera. Imagine the possibilities! They ARE salads, now aren't they? They DO contain more calories, but not as many as an entire entrée.

Remember, this is YOUR GAME, YOUR RULES.

22.   HAVE A SOUP DAY

For years and years soup has always been the mainstay on any dieting plan. They're readily available in packages, jars, or cans. They're very easy to throw together at home. Most of the ingredients can often be found in your cupboards and refrigerator.

This is one crutch you may think is impossible to use as far as breakfast is concerned. Who would ever have soup for breakfast? People do have tomato juice as a breakfast beverage, don't they? Sure they do. And you can have as much as you want. You didn't promise to have half-portions for the day, did you? Actually, you may have soup for breakfast, lunch, or dinner.

Your soups don't have to be consommés either. They can be as hearty as you want them to be. You make the rules –you adhere to them. I'd be willing to bet, however, that because you are playing these games to lose weight, you probably won't take as much leeway as you could. You want to stay within the boundaries of the program.

23.   HAVE A LIQUID DAY

You can start your day using this crutch with your breakfast beverage — tomato, cranberry, pineapple, orange, guava – whatever you desire – how much you desire – how often you desire.

Having nothing but liquids all day is very easy to accomplish. You may drink any food which can be changed into a liquid form, at any time of day – all day long.

Your blender or food processor will come into play constantly. You may indulge in any kind of liquids – juices, sodas, even ice cream sodas or milkshakes. It's up to you.

Again, the possibilities are endless and you're having fun while sticking to the program. You're still playing the game.

This crutch is actually the easiest of them all to implement because the stomach remains full and you never experience hunger pains. Having different flavors of drinks will keep you from becoming bored.

24. EAT ONLY FRUITS AND VEGETABLES

I'm certain you've heard about the benefits of eating six to eight fruits and vegetables daily. Of course, that's when they're eaten in conjunction with the other food groups. The dark green, leafy vegetables are considered to be the most beneficial, however, any kind of vegetable has it's own, unique quality.

You certainly wouldn't (or shouldn't) eat only fruits and vegetables every day of your life. However, doing so for one day would expend a significant amount of calories, to say nothing of eliminating fats from your diet.

All of us do try to do the right thing all of the time but there are times when we just don't have the will power. That's where this plan comes into play. We ask for help— for will power from the One we worship. We make our promise. We choose our crutch for the day. We stick to our promise every time we feel our resolve weakening.

25. ENJOY A GRAZING DAY

Imagine eating whatever you want at any time of day that suits your fancy. Sounds delicious, yes? Well, you can. From the time you get out of bed to the time you go to sleep at night, you may eat all day long. You snack whenever you want to. You won't consume your three complete, heavy meals.

I'm willing to bet the farm that you won't overindulge because you know you are implementing this crutch in order to lose weight. Why would you gorge yourself with humungous amounts while grazing? It would be a stupid thing to do.

Grazing would be even more effective if you ate only when you're hungry. This would really cut down on your calories for the day. It may be a little more difficult to accomplish, but just keep reminding yourself that tomorrow's another day. It's another day when you can choose a crutch that you find easier to live with. This thought alone will help to keep you on track. Remember, it's ONE DAY AT A TIME.

26. PERUSE ALL FOOD LABELS

One of the easiest ways to lose weight is to KNOW WHAT YOU'RE EATING. If you take the time to read the nutrition labels on all of the foods before you purchase them, you undoubtedly won't choose those which have the larger amounts of fats or calories. I know there have been countless times that I have made another choice of a particular food which I had planned on purchasing after I read (and was shocked at) how many calories and/or grams of fat it contained.

You think that canned fruits in their own juices just don't taste as good as those in heavy syrup. Believe me, a few samplings of fruits in their own juice will convince you that they taste as good as the other. You'll probably decide that the syrupy ones are actually disgustingly sweet, and you will seek out the "Less Fat" and "Lite" labels which are cropping up more and more. Some of these foods can also be used in cooking without any detection whatsoever. Consequently, you're losing calories just by substitution. How easy is that?

27.   COUNT EVERY CALORIE

Today you will choose this crutch and make your promise to count each and every calorie that is in every piece of food you put into your mouth.   It's a very simple thing to do, considering all of the diet booklets there are out there which list the amount of calories in every food imaginable.   They are clearly listed by either pieces, ounces, or serving sizes.

First you need to determine the acceptable total of calories which are allowed daily to unable your body to lose weight.   This, too, is easily ascertained by consulting the numerous health books on the subject.

Once you start eating you need to jot down every calorie you consume during the entire day.   That means you list your breakfast, any mid-morning snack, your lunch, afternoon snacks, dinner, and bedtime snack.   It's also necessary to keep a running total all day long. You'll need to keep track of each and every calorie or you may reach your daily limit by mid-day.   You wouldn't want to have to stop eating by lunch time, would you?

28. COUNT EVERY
GRAM OF FAT

40 grams of fat is considered the limit an average person should consume daily – even when they're not trying to lose weight.

Again, you will need to document each gram of fat you swallow from breakfast to dinner, including any between-meal snacks you might eat at any time during the day or evening. Once more, you will need to read labels on all the foods you use today.

I would suggest that you don't use this crutch immediately after using the Count Every Calorie crutch. You'll find yourself getting bored with all that counting and documenting and you may lose interest in the program itself. Instead, choose a crutch that you really find easy to live with.

If you do monitor your grams of fat I guarantee that once you become aware of how many grams each food contains you'll select those foods which are low in fat over those which are high.

29. EAT <u>ONLY ONE</u> BETWEEN MEAL SNACK

This crutch is a cousin to the Half Portions one— only a little bit more extreme. It is especially advantageous to the chronic munchers, and they are legion.

If you are one of those munchers and <u>must</u> eat between meals, promise to eat only ONE piece of your chosen snack. Yes, I do mean only ONE cookie, only ONE cracker, only ONE grape, only ONE peanut — only ONE of whatever.

Of course, this also means that you're allowed to have only ONE <u>large</u> candy bar. You see how this program works? It may seem a little ludicrous but it's a game, after all. It's a game and you're the one playing it. You're the one who's making the rules. You know that you can have that large candy bar because it IS only ONE. You know you <u>can</u>, but you most likely <u>won't</u> because you know it will set back your progress and because it's entirely up to you how quickly you want to reach your ultimate weight loss goal.

30.   SKIP A MEAL

Did I say "skip a meal"? Yes, that's what I said. Unorthodox? Of course. Unheard of? Yes. Every nutritionist in the world worth his weight in salt will tell you that this is an extremely unhealthy course of action.

However, if you implement this crutch just once in a very great while, during the course of the program, to help you keep on playing the losing game, why not? Additionally, if you skipped your lunch and went for a walk instead, you'd derive twice the benefits from this crutch. You'd be eliminating calories and exercising off any calories you gained from your previous meal.

The most efficient use of this crutch would be to skip your dinner. It won't be the easiest thing to do because dinner is usually the most enjoyable meal of the day. Everyone knows that you should eat the last meal of the day as early as possible to be able to work off most of the calories before retiring.   If you had NOTHING to eat for your last meal of the day you would not need to worry about them.

31. HAVE ONLY ONE
MEAL TODAY

This is a crutch which is comparable to skipping a meal. The obvious difference is that instead of having two meals for the day, you will indulge in only one. This will decrease your caloric intake by two-thirds from a normal three meal day. It won't be as difficult to do as you think, either. All you need to do is to fill your stomach with liquids during the other two meal times.

32. USE A COMBINATION OF CRUTCHES

Using two or three crutches in one day such as eating only one of anything, counting every calorie, skipping a meal, or any other combination, would really expend a substantial amount of calories in one day. It may be a little difficult to remember each crutch, but keeping your note accessible all day will help you. You also need to be an extremely disciplined person, but perhaps you <u>are</u> that sort of person. Congratulations!

33. ABOUT YOUR FAMILY

It just occurred to me that while I have been presenting all of these crutches for you to choose each day — and there will be more — I haven't even touched on the fact that you probably are not a single person living alone. You probably have a family that you need to take into consideration when you plan a diet regimen.

You most likely have surmised by now that I am a single woman (actually widowed) in my later years of life. You're thinking that it's effortless for me to make all the rules I want because they don't affect anyone else. That's only partially true. It's easier in one respect, but more difficult in another. I CAN eat whatever I want, WHENEVER I want. True, this is an asset, however, it's also a liability. The fact that I can eat whatever suits my fancy, at whatever time of day I opt for, makes it easier to throw caution to the winds. If I had someone else to consider, I would need to be more circumspect in choosing healthy foods for each and every meal.

Enlist your family's participation. If the rest of your household would also like to lose weight (or trim down a bit), it will be fun for all of you to choose a particular crutch for the day. When you all go off to work or school you can all use the honor system. Expecting your children to do so is teaching them to uphold their family's moral code. Having your entire family participate in the program will facilitate your achieving your goal. It will also make it infinitely easier to implement many of the crutches. When you return home you certainly won't have any trouble communicating about the pressures any of you might have experienced while keeping the promise for the day.

This program also brings about family togetherness. Can any other diet plan say the same? As you already know, good communication between partners and/or family members is the primary requisite for a happy life. My husband and I were very compatible and had no trouble communicating. Nevertheless, it took me quite a while to get my husband into the program with me. My children were already grown and out of the house. When I finally succeeded to convince him to take the plunge, he really got into it. He would say "okay kiddo, what are we giving up today?" We'd have a good laugh and then we'd both decide which food we were going to eliminate that day, or even if we were going to play that day at all. Of course, he was a great guy and very easy to live with, but even a more difficult spouse can be won over with a little determination and work.

Almost every crutch in the program is adaptable to both individual and/or family use. Having your entire household participate will make it easier for you to accomplish your own goal. You will be able to eat the same meal as they.

It will also give you more incentive not to sample the food while you're preparing their meals. In addition, If you realize that you are being a role model for your family, you will become more committed to eat slowly, eat only half-portions, chew your food eight times before swallowing, drink a full glass of water before each meal, etc. etc. Your legacy becomes "do as I do".

34. CREATE A COMPLETE MEAL FROM YOUR FAVORITE FOOD

Remember when you were a child and couldn't get enough of your favorite food? It could have been peanut butter and jelly sandwiches. Your mother said another kind of sandwich could never pass your lips. The only cereal you would eat was Cheerios, or maybe Cocoa Puffs. The only fruit you would touch would be a banana.

Maybe you still feel the same way. Even as an adult you have a certain food that appeals to you more than others. Well, you can have a day of eating just your favorite food...for breakfast, lunch, and dinner. Beyond the shadow of a doubt, you won't crave it as much from then on. If you're smart, though, you'll use the half-portion crutch in conjunction with it.

Be careful of using this crutch too often. It shouldn't be used more than once a month because you could consume a large amount of fats and calories if your favorite food is laden with them.

Maybe this crutch sounds foolish to you. Maybe several of them do. Perhaps you're right. Perhaps some of them <u>are</u> silly, even ludicrous, but I told you in the beginning that this program was going to be FUN to participate in. You may think you're too sophisticated to employ some of them. It's up to you. You can either take pride in your cultured, Ivy-League overweight façade or you can employ the silly crutches, participate in the program and take pride in your new, svelte body.

Every crutch you use throughout each day keeps you interested regardless of how silly it might seem. If you keep at it you'll have the last laugh and to stay focused on your ultimate goal to lose those unwanted pounds, all you need to do is review the list of crutches, (which is Crutch No. 45 discussed on Page 65), choose one for the day, and keep losing weight. ONE DAY AT A TIME. There are those magic words again. Keep them in your mind constantly.

35.   UTILIZE ANY OLD DIET

Remember all of the diet plans we mentioned in the first paragraph? I'm positive you know of even many more, some you've read about, heard about, or even tried yourself.

Would you believe that you can put one or more of them to use as part of this program?

Well, you can.

The way you approached those diets in the past was to attempt to adhere to them for a week, a month, or even more challenging, you would think about sticking to them indefinitely. You found you just couldn't do it. It was too difficult— almost impossible. You just didn't like the monotony of the diet, or you didn't feel satisfied with the amount of food you were allowed to have. You quit. Now you can try to make them work for you.

Here's what you do. You make one of these diets your crutch for the day. You will undoubtedly lose a little bit of weight and you can add this to your accumulative weight loss.

Again remember, it's ONE DAY AT A TIME.

36. HAVE A "FATLESS" DAY

This crutch is one which everyone should try to do whether or not they participate in this program. It's almost imperative to do so if a person has any history of heart problems in their family or in their own life. Fat not only is the worse ingredient you can put into your body for health reasons, it's the worse thing you can ingest if you are trying to achieve a svelte, shapely figure.

To utilize this crutch read every nutrition label on each and every food you put into your mouth today, from your breakfast beverage and cereal to the dessert at your evening meal, and choose the ones with no fat.

37.   HAVE A FISH DAY

If you're a seafood lover this will be easy. It will also be extremely effective because we all know how few calories and fat it contains (providing it's prepared without any fat or served without any butter).

38. GIVE YOURSELF A "FREE" DAY

No matter what kind of regimen you are a part of, whether it be a diet or a study of any kind, you need to be able to take a day off now and then. So it is with this program. Take a day off and throw caution to the winds. It won't cause you to undo all the progress you've already made, and it will be emotionally beneficial to you. I guarantee that if you have already participated in this program for any length of time, you have conditioned yourself to eat in moderation. Even though you're taking a day off you won't overindulge yourself. You've already trained yourself NOT TO.

39. CHOOSE AN EXTREMELY DIFFICULT CRUTCH

Rise to the occasion and challenge yourself. It'll certainly build your character and give you a great feeling of accomplish-ment, especially if you choose to do this after you've indulged yourself in a "Free Day".

40. PLACE A "FAT" MAGNET
ON YOUR REFRIGERATOR

I have a cute little pig that monitors my caloric intake each time I approach the refrigerator. I also have a note on it which reads "A MOMENT ON THE LIPS, FOREVER ON THE HIPS". Every little reminder helps. There are times when I choose to ignore the warnings but, when my eyes do make contact they are like strings around my finger to keep me focused on what I'm trying to do — lose weight.

You are especially fortunate if you have a special event you wish to attend in the near future. It will give you that extra incentive you need to stick to your resolve to lose weight. You can rationalize that you'll play the game just long enough to get into that special outfit for that important event. Then you'll be off the hook! However, let me tell you that once you have reached that goal, and realize how easy it was to accomplish it, you'll want to continue playing the games to <u>maintain</u> your weight loss.

Just remember one thing. If you're going to play the game and be successful at it, you need to be honest with yourself. For example, if you're not particularly fond of certain foods, such as cheese, bacon, sweets, or whatever, don't use them as one of the crutches. Quite clearly, you're only defeating your purpose. What's the point?

The most important factor in losing weight, and getting your body in shape, is to make it the very first priority in your life. Think of improving your health and sculpting your body when you first awaken in the morning. Think of it when you make your choice of food you are going to eliminate for the day. Think of it when you measure out a half-portion at every meal. Think of it when you perform your daily exercises.

In other words, make keeping your body healthy the most important thing in your life — because it is. Keep it in your mind constantly, make it the very first priority in your life and protect it with every means at your disposal.

41. SHARE YOUR
RESTAURANT MEAL

In today's society it seems that all restaurants are in competition with each other to determine who can pile on the most food. This is certainly evident in the physiques of their clientele. Simply take a count of the obese (or nearly obese) patrons the next time you go out to eat. America is having a problem — an obesity problem. You need to help yourself — and I don't mean to the food. The restaurants obviously won't help you.

When people describe their visit to a restaurant they don't critique the quality of the food. They expound on the <u>quantity.</u> When my daughter and I go out to eat, we SHARE a meal. Most restaurants will accommodate us by giving us a second plate, but once in a while they will impose a $1.00 sharing plate charge. This is a small price to pay to avoid overeating.

There is one particular restaurant in our area which serves such gigantic portions that even though we share a meal we still take home "doggie bags". Needless to say, neither of us owns a dog. I, personally, can have two more meals from the leftovers. When I dine alone, I still take a doggie bag home. It's not that I

<u>couldn't</u> eat the entire meal, because I have a ravenous appetite and have no trouble at all scoffing up whatever is placed on my plate.

Whenever I go to a restaurant alone I also use the Half-Portion Crutch to help me stomach partially with a glass of water at the beginning of the meal. Then I eat a couple of rolls (which is really no sacrifice for me because I love rolls). When the entrée is served I find myself feeling very satisfied with only half of it. I ask to have the remainder packed up which allows me to have another half-portion meal the next day without any effort on my part at all.

Do you see how you can adapt this program to your personal needs? As I told you before, YOU make the rules. That's what makes it so very interesting and it's what keeps you on track. That's why it is so successful. Before you know it, you've reached your goal. And it was so easy!

42. AVOID FAST FOOD RESTAURANTS

like the plague. Just about any restaurant presents a challenge to a dieter. A fast food restaurant is definitely at the top of that list. Virtually every item on the menu is loaded with fats and carbohydrates — to say nothing of being loaded with cholesterol.

BUT HOLD THE PHONE! This remarkable program allows you to indulge yourself with a fast food product, even a greasy gigantic cheeseburger — if you feel you just can't live another day without one. Only ONE.

Again, YOU'RE the one playing the game and making the rules. There is only one stipulation (actually three) to this crutch. All you need to do after you've satisfied your sinful craving is to vow to use <u>two crutches</u> the next day to make up for your transgression. You must also promise not to frequent another fast food restaurant for a long, long, long time to come. Maybe never.

43.   ABSTAIN FROM FOOD THE ENTIRE DAY OF A PARTY

When you know you are going to be tempted with wonderful food at a dinner party or wedding, or with luscious hors d'oeuvre at a pre-dinner gathering, doesn't it make sense to prepare for it? You bet. If you merely drink beverages all day long, you can attend the affair with a carefree heart. You will enjoy the social part of the gathering that much more.

44. STATION YOURSELF AWAY FROM THE REFRESHMENT TABLE

After you have taken a small (or at least reasonable) portion of hors d'oeuvre, take your plate and yourself into another room. After your first helping it's inevitable that your taste buds will be awakened and it's much too easy to replenish the food if you're standing only an arm's length from it.

In another room you can converse with the people who are not positioning themselves in front of the tempting, overabundant buffet.

45. CONSULT TABLE OF CONTENTS

In order to make your task easier and to help you stay on track, consult the Table of Contents every morning to review all of the available crutches. Choose one for the day, make your pledge to your Supreme Being, write it down on a piece of note paper and keep it with you for the entire day as a constant reminder. More than just a reminder, it will be a powerful motivator as you go through your day.

Hopefully, you will be strong enough that nothing — none of your daily activities — will keep you from participating in the program. If, by chance, you DO lose sight of your goal at one time or another and skip a day or two, or even a week or two, just return to it as you possibly can.

Everyone slips off the wagon at one time or another. We're only human. Don't beat yourself up over it. Just start again. Remember, if at first you don't succeed, try try again.

46.   SET A REALISTIC GOAL

If you have 50 pounds or more to lose, don't tell yourself that you'll do it in a month. You won't. Nobody can. Even if by some miracle they could, whatever method they used would be dangerous to their health. As I am writing this, a pharmaceutical company is testing a new drug to help us lose weight. They said "it's a drug that stops you from eating a little bit sooner". DUH! Isn't that our "Eat Half Portions" crutch? Let's stick to our ONE DAY AT A TIME drugless program.

The Alcoholics Anonymous group is very successful eliciting that philosophy, and so it is with this program. Their prayer:

> God grant me the serenity
> To accept the things I cannot change,
> <u>Courage to change the things I can</u>, and
> Wisdom to know the difference

has provided me with guidance and strength throughout my lifetime and it has never let me down – never. I have a large, framed copy of it in my den as a constant inspiration.

47. USE THE BUDDY SYSTEM

Whenever we try any new diet it always helps if we have someone to share it with. If you have a friend who also wants to lose weight (and who doesn't?) explain the program to them and I'm sure they will find it completely intriguing. Everyone is always eager to hear about a different diet, especially one which is so simple and foolproof. They will be motivated to at least <u>try</u> another new one. They'll think "maybe this one will work". They're going to be surprised when it does.

Make plans for the two of you to use the same crutch every day for at least a week, or better still for a month. Each of you decides together which food to eliminate for the day or which reducing crutch to use. At the end of the time agreed upon, compare your rewarding losses of weight.

The benefit of employing the Buddy System is that not only does it give you more incentives and motivation, you also have the opportunity to call him/her if you're ever tempted to stray from your chosen path.

48.   TRY TO FIT INTO
AN OLD PAIR OF JEANS

There is nothing more frustrating than trying to put on an outfit and discover that it doesn't fit.   You relegate it to the farthest corner in your most remote closet in the house. You tell yourself that you ARE going to go on a diet and that you ARE going to fit into it again. Okay, that was about a year ago.

Now that you've decided to give this program a chance to take off the pounds, try to get those jeans on again.   They'll be a great motivator.   Keep trying them on periodically during the process.   If you'd rather wait a couple of weeks in between fittings — fine. You only need to keep a mental picture of yourself in that outfit while you're using your daily crutches.   Keep it in your mind every time you reach for any food at all.

They say a picture is worth a thousand words.   In this case it's worth at least a hundred calories — maybe even a thousand. The amount depends on the effort you put into the program. YOU call the shots.

49. SHOP THE MALL – TO TRY, NOT TO BUY

Like trying to fit into a pair of tight jeans, there is no more effective motivation to go on a diet than viewing yourself in a three-way mirror in a dress boutique at the mall. Seeing yourself in an outfit which makes you look like a stuffed sausage is enough to make you never want to eat another morsel in your lifetime.

Go shopping and try on outfits in a size that is the one you would <u>like</u> to fit into – if you can get into it. Stand in front of that merciless mirror. Be extremely critical. Peruse every roll and bulge. Try on several outfits (or attempt to).

I guarantee that after you check out all the lovely new styles and by the time you leave the mall, your resolve to lose weight will be stronger than ever. You won't even want to wait for the next day to start losing the calories which will allow you to put on those beautiful outfits. You may even use one of the crutches for the remainder of your shopping day

You have undoubtedly heard of all of these aforementioned crutches at one time or another, but just hearing about them is not the same as putting them into practice. You require constant motivation to make them work – motivation you receive from making your pledges to your Supreme Being. By now you know that this program teaches you how to accomplish this

You now also have more than enough crutches to use a different one each day for over a month. Interesting? You bet. Boring? Hardly. Fun? Of course. NOW JUST DO IT!

EXERCISE –
AN ESSENTIAL COMPONENT

You <u>could</u> lose weight by implementing the aids and crutches alone, but this program is also an overall health program, so another important vow you need to make to your God is to promise to EXERCISE DAILY. Exercise not only trims your figure – it keeps you healthy. Of course, you already know that, but you need the extra incentive you receive when you promise Him that you <u>will</u> exercise.

When you have performed only twelve repetitions of an exercise for your head, neck, shoulders, arms, waist, stomach, hips, legs, ankles and feet, you will have stretched and toned every part of your body in approximately a mere twelve minutes. ONLY 12 MINUTES!

Even if after a late evening of dancing, working, or just watching late night television, you really hate the thought of exercising the next morning, and you tell yourself that just for today you'll skip the exercise routine— DON'T. It has been proven that ENERGY CREATES ENERGY. Force yourself to do the bare minimum of repetitions, maybe only two or three. Subsequently you will find yourself doing even more reps and when you have awakened every part of your body, you have increased your vitality, enabling you to complete your daily tasks. If you want to stop at the two or three repetitions, you'll still increase the level of vitality that you had before you started exercising.

Continually picture yourself as a trim and svelte beauty and you will be more than willing, even anxious, to exercise. Your good health is the primary reason for exercising. Improving your figure is an extra bonus.

This is a new day. Rejoice in it! You have been given another day — another opportunity — to improve your health, to sculpt your body, to improve your mind, to care for your family — to LIVE.

YOU know which part of your body needs the most attention. While you are performing your daily dozen, choose a spot exercise for that particular body part and do ten extra reps. My stomach has always been my biggest problem so I daily do ten extra reps of stomach crunches. In addition, I also do an isometric exercise whenever I'm driving my car. Actually, It's not while I'm <u>driving</u>, it's while I'm stopped for a stop sign or traffic light. I keep my stomach muscles contracted during the time I'm waiting for the light to change or for my turn to proceed through the intersection. It took quite a while for me to train myself to remember to do the stomach isometric every time I applied the brake, but I now find myself doing it automatically. It has become a habit. A good habit.

LOOK FORWARD TO YOUR DAILY EXERCISES. Don't think of them as a chore. Think of how very important it is to keep every part of your body as supple as possible to keep you as healthy as you can be, to be able to complete your daily obligations.

Exercise also attributes to calories expended. For every pound of muscle you bring into your body you burn an extra 35 to 50 calories a day. The more muscle you build, the more calories you expend. Now, that's a plus if there ever was one!

The exercises I am presenting in this book are the very minimal. You, yourself, undoubtedly know of numerous others which you may certainly add to the required daily dozen. You probably will. Exercising is contagious. The more you do, the more you want to do. It makes you feel good. Why wouldn't you want more?

The exercising section of this program is as simple as the food section. It uses the identical principle. You promise your God that you <u>will</u> exercise every day. You make that promise when you choose your crutch for the day. There might be a day when it's impossible for you to honor your obligation. For instance, you may be leaving on a trip at 4:00 A.M. and, no way could you fit in your exercising. Well, you're excused. You may not even be able to fit it in the next day, or even for the next week. However, when you return to your normal way of living, you will make and keep your promise again.

You know what you have to do. You know how to do it. Let's get exercising!!

EYES – There are very few (hardly any) exercise programs which include exercises for the eyes. I wonder why. You wouldn't be able to do any visual chores if you couldn't see. It isn't as if these exercises are going to bring back anyone's sight, but exercising the eye muscles do help to keep your eyesight strong.

Sit or stand erect. Look up and hold for 5 seconds. Look down and hold for 5 seconds. Look to the right and hold for 5 seconds. Look to the left and hold for 5 seconds. Repeat the entire exercise 10 times.

HEAD & NECK: Without keeping your head and neck flexible you wouldn't even be able to drive a car safely. It would be difficult to look behind you before putting it into reverse. It seems like a simple function of your body, but it certainly isn't for someone who is unable to do it.

Sit or stand erect. Turn your head as far to the right as is comfortable, back to the center, and then to the right. Repeat 12 times.

Sit or stand erect. Drop your chin to your chest. Roll it up to your left, then to the right. Repeat 12 times. Do not roll your head to the back.

SHOULDERS – You want to play ball with your children (or grandchildren), you want to mow the lawn, hang curtains, play golf or tennis, row a boat, or just accomplish whatever activity you need (or want) to do. You need flexible shoulders.

Stand erect. Simply <u>slowly</u> rotate your shoulders forward and back, back and forward twelve times.

Stand with feet approximately one foot apart. Let your arms hang down and clasp your fingers behind your back. Raise your shoulders up and rotate them to the back. Stretch back and hold the position for five seconds. Repeat twelve times.

ARMS — Strong arms will permit you to push your toddler on a swing, or to have a game of hoops with your teenager. Your arms will cease to flutter when you wear that strapless gown to your next formal affair

Sit on a chair with your back straight holding a 1 to 5 lb. weight above your head. With your opposite hand on your triceps, bend your arm down behind you, keeping your elbow near your head. Repeat 10 times, then switch arms.

FINGERS – It's almost impossible to imagine how limited your activities would be without the complete use of your fingers. You would be unable to maneuver kitchen utensils, handle a hammer or screw driver, use a computer, play the piano, et cetera, et cetera. In essence, you could hardly do anything at all if your fingers didn't function.

Manipulating your fingers helps to both prevent and ease the pain of existing arthritis. I have been doing this exercise for years. I think I learned about it from a Yoga book I had read.

Extend your hands in front of you with palms down. Stretch each digit apart from each other, one at a time, as far as you possibly can. Stretch and hold until it is slightly painful.

Stretch each finger and thumb upward one at a time. Again, hold it until almost painful.

Now curl each digit down, one at a time, one knuckle at a time until you form fists. This needs to be performed only once — but very slowly.

WAIST – A slim waist is the goal of almost every woman in the world with the exception of the few who have one. But they most likely have other problems with their bodies which are not as discernible. Nobody – no body – is perfect. At least almost nobody.

To get back to the waist, picture your new figure in that form-fitting, slinky cocktail dress you'll be wearing on that cruise, or that great, sexy fitted dress you bought for that special wedding, or that cute shorts and top ensemble you're going to wear to your daughter's school picnic.

Stand erect with your feet approximately one foot apart and your hands at the sides of your waist. Twist slowly to the left, bending your right knee until you are facing the back and then around to the right, bending your left knee until you are facing the back. End the exercise facing front. Repeat 10 times.

Keep standing erect with feet apart. Reach up with your right arm. Slowly bend over to the left as far as possible, sliding your left hand down your left leg. Repeat on the other side. Do ten repetitions.

BACK – If you have ever been to a chiropractor you know that they have different kinds of equipment to help them with their therapy. One of these pieces of equipment is a flat table with rollers built in which massage your back one vertebra at a time. You can experience this same therapy at home. If you are presently having stiffness in your back, this exercise will loosen it up. If you don't, it will keep your back muscles supple enough to prevent any back pain.

Lie on your back. Bring your knees to your chest. Clasp your fingers together under your knees. Raise your back up and roll back and forth.

Another variation: Lie on your back. Bring your knees to your chest. Cross your feet at the ankles. Grasp your right toes with your left hand and your left toes with your right hand. Raise your back up and roll back and forth. Repeat as many times as you like. It will feel so good to have your back massaged that you'll do more reps than I could ever suggest.

DERRIERE – This exercise will not only give you a firmer derriere and make you look great in your new slacks. Medically, it will strengthen your bladder muscles to help ward off incontinence in the future.

Lie on the floor with your knees bent. Keep your feet flat on the floor and hands next to your body with palms down. Slowly lift your hips off the floor until your chest, hips and knees are in one line. Squeeze your buttocks together, contracting the muscles, and hold for 3 seconds. Lower your spine to the floor, one vertebra at a time. Repeat 10 times.

STOMACH – This is probably the part of the body that most people complain about, men as well as women. The most effective exercises are crunches and sit-ups. I already told you about my special "driving exercise".

Lie on your back with your knees bent, your legs together, your feet stretched out and elevated. Lift your head and shoulders off the floor. Extend your arms out straight, next to your legs. Pump your arms forward and back, keeping your abdominal muscles firm as you count to 25. Repeat 10 times.

HIPS – You saw an adorable knit dress at the mall but you didn't even try it on because you knew it would reveal every lump and roll on your hips. Take heart. If you pay special attention and focus your exercising efforts on your hips, you'll get into that dress before you know it. You'll be fighting that worn out cliché which states "a moment on the lips, forever on the hips".

Standing tall with feet about two feet apart, slowly slide your right hand down your right leg as far as you possibly can. Hold the position for 3 seconds. Do not bounce. Come up and repeat on the left side. Do 10 reps.

Lie down on the floor on your left side. Extend your left arm straight up, resting your head on it. Place your right hand in front of you for support. Now lift your legs off the floor and "bicycle" 25 times. You will be literally "rubbing the fat off your hips". Repeat on right side.

LEGS — The contour of a person's legs is very difficult to change, however, there are exercises which can reduce the fat which has accumulated over the years. You don't have to wear slacks or floor length skirts for the rest of your life. As I said before, if there is any special part of your body that you want to change, make an extra effort to zero in on the exercises that will correct the problem. There are many exercises which focus on the legs. Here are just two of them:

To firm up your calves. Stand with your feet close together. Contract your calf muscles, pulling them in together as tight as you can. Repeat 10 times.

Lie on your left side, your body raised at the waist, resting your weight on your left arm which is bent at the elbow. Keep your right hand in front of you for support. Lift your right leg about six inches off the floor. Keeping your right leg stiff and steady, lift and lower your bottom leg (the left one) 10 times. Switch sides and repeat 10 times. Do four repetitions.

FEET – As far as I'm concerned, exercising my feet is absolutely imperative. For me, it's paramount because my very first love in life (second only to my children and grandchildren) is ballroom dancing. Then comes tap dancing. Can you see why exercising my feet is so important to me? Even if I have no time at all to do the entire exercise regimen (which very seldom happens, because I start my day with the exercises) I would never think of not performing the ones that keep my feet healthy.

Sit on the floor supporting yourself with your hands at your sides. Flex and point each foot twenty times. You can either use the same foot for all twenty reps, or you can alternate each foot twenty times.

Remaining seated, flex and rotate each foot slowly for at least 12 times.

Standing up with your feet six inches apart, slowly raise your body up onto your toes and lower it back onto your heels. Repeat 10 times.

EACH PART OF YOUR BODY
HAS BEEN EXERCISED

Now, how long did that take you? Approximately twelve to fifteen minutes. Fifteen minutes out of twenty-four hours! Don't tell me (or yourself) that you can't devote fifteen minutes a day to keeping (or making) yourself healthy.

After you have performed the routine several times and become familiar with it, it won't even take that long. It's easy enough to remember because it goes from head to toe. You'll perform each exercise automatically and enjoy doing it.

EXERCISE THROUGHOUT THE DAY

USE CLEANING YOUR HOUSE TO EXERCISE. Dusting, vacuuming, scouring the tub, washing windows — all these cleaning chores can aid you in sculpting your body and maintaining your good health. Just STRETCH your arms further than necessary, REACH high above your head while dusting high places, BEND from the waist when retrieving something from the floor, TWIST from side to side while vacuuming. Make every movement

COUNT. Believe me, you won't need to join a gym, and your house will sparkle.

PERFORM A SPECIFIC SPOT EXERCISE EVERY HOUR. You can perform a spot exercise every hour whether you're at home, in the car, or at work. You just need to choose one that is not obvious to anyone else.

Contracting the stomach muscles can be done discreetly. Foot exercises can be done under your desk. Many of them can be performed out of the home and the others can be done in the privacy of your home. The point here is to execute an exercise every hour.

I could go on and on, ad infinitum, about the benefits of exercise, but you know what I'm getting at. It doesn't take a Washington attorney or a neuro-surgeon to comprehend. In a nutshell, everyone MUST exercise to maintain a healthy body, to say nothing of being able to achieve the figure they have always admired. I guarantee that if you focus on these advantages you will look forward to your daily exercises.

I cannot stress too strongly that you MUST make exercising your very first priority. You must understand clearly, without a shadow of a doubt, that exercising is not just an activity you fit in between your other daily tasks. It is the

<u>most important</u> activity you will perform on any given day.

You wouldn't be able to accomplish any task at all if you were not physically capable of doing so, if your body would rebel at almost any movement. Consequently, doesn't it make sense to assure yourself that you <u>will</u> be able to do so by just performing a few simple, isometric or aerobic movements?

It's imperative that, along with your exercises, you also make YOU your first priority. You must put yourself first — even before your family. This may sound selfish to you but, in truth, it isn't. By keeping your body fit and healthy you are physically able to look after your family's needs. You would not be capable to care for them if you were incapacitated in any way.

At the risk of my being redundant, the only single way of accomplishing this is to EXERCISE.

After an accident, a stroke, or any other debilitating illness, and after the surgery is performed and the drugs are utilized, you know that doctors prescribe physical therapy to restore flexibility to weakened or atrophied muscles.

Doesn't it make sense, then, to perform the physical therapy <u>before</u> the illness or accident? Exercising is the same as having physical therapy. The only difference is that you, yourself, are the physical therapist.

A few years ago I had a recurring bout with bursitis in my left elbow. The pain was severe enough for me to consult an orthopedist. That action, in itself, added to my pain because I avoid going to a doctor's office as much as possible except for yearly checkups.

He injected cortisone into the area. Miracle of miracles! The pain disappeared! I was pain free for several months, but my paradise was short-lived. Again the pain reared its ugly head. Again I went to the doctor's office. Again I got a shot of cortisone. This time, however, the pain-free period was of a much shorter duration than the previous time.

When I found myself in the doctor's office for the third time, he told me I had two more options other than the cortisone (which was losing its effectiveness). I could elect to have surgery or I could come in for a series of physical therapy. As far as I was concerned, the surgery was not an option. I asked what the physical therapy would entail. He informed me that a physical therapist would manipulate the area over several weeks until the pain subsided.

I decided to research my condition to find out if I had anything in my own power to rid myself of the persistent pain. I delved into as many resources as were possible. Most of the information available pertained to bursitis in the shoulder area. I finally found a source relating to the elbow which prescribed a very simple exercise. The bursitis being in my left elbow, all I needed to do was to hold out my left arm and rub the elbow with the index and middle fingers of my right hand.

The only difficult part of the therapy was that the elbow needed to be manipulated for long periods of time, several times a day. Because I was determined to rid myself of the pain, I rubbed my elbow almost constantly. My tenacity paid off. After a couple of weeks the pain subsided substantially. It wasn't too much longer that the pain was almost gone entirely.

For several months, whenever I felt any feeling of the bursitis returning, no matter how slight, I would perform the therapy again. I have not had any recurrence of the condition for several years now.

To further sing the praises of exercise, I want to tell you about an 85 year old man who, at the age of 81, woke up one morning unable to walk. He was admitted to the hospital, went through surgery, and left the hospital in a wheelchair. The prognosis was not very promising. This was especially devastating to him since he had been a ballroom dance instructor and had been dancing up to the day he was stricken with the malady. His feelings were that if he couldn't dance he really didn't care much whether he lived or died. Dancing <u>WAS</u> his life. He was determined he would dance again. Armed with this determination and positive attitude, he disciplined himself to faithfully exercise his legs and feet daily

After over a year of exercising he was able to walk, first with the aid of a walker and then with a cane. He attended dances where at first he was only able to watch, but then after a period of time he was able to execute the steps to a slow waltz and a slow foxtrot. He is now capable of performing every form of dance from the waltz to the swing and all of the Latin dances as well. Not only would this be a remarkable fete for a younger man, the fact that he is 85 years old is overwhelming testimony to the powers of a positive attitude and EXERCISE.

My daughter has her own philosophy of keeping trim and healthy. She says it's so simple, it's ludicrous. She lives by the theory that you should EAT LESS, EXERCISE MORE. She says that one of these days she's going to write a book containing only those four words. "EAT LESS, EXERCISE MORE".

Quite clearly, this is a tried and true philosophy, but most people are not disciplined enough to follow through without outside help.

By using this program, <u>you</u> can receive all of the help you need.

I need to confess to you that it wasn't easy for me to devise this program. There were many pitfalls. I had three strikes against me before I even started.

First of all, I LOVE TO COOK. I can curl up and read a cook book like other people read a novel. There's nothing I enjoy better than to find a new recipe — especially in a gourmet cook book. I love to shop for the ingredients. I really revel in the processes of chopping, sautéing, mixing, and executing all of the intriguing steps which go into creating a gourmet meal. Can you possibly understand what the art of cooking and baking means to me?

Secondly, I LOVE TO EAT. I have a burly truck driver's appetite in my five foot frame. When I was employed by a firm which had its own cafeteria, everyone in the food line couldn't help but remark about the amount of food I put on my tray. And I ate every bit of what I took. There was a lot of good natured kidding at our table. That was when I was younger and the calories didn't show up as quickly as they do now.

Thirdly, I LOVE TO GO TO RESTAURANTS. I enjoy all types of restaurants and all types of foods from hamburgers to pheasant under glass. I can't think of one food that I wouldn't at least sample. If I don't have a friend (or my daughter) to accompany me to a lunch or dinner out, I think nothing of going by myself.

Besides the three strikes against me there is another hazard in my life that I have to contend with while trying to lose weight. My working hours are from 3:00 to 8:00 P.M., making my normal dinner time between 8:30 and 9:00 P.M.

It's common knowledge that the easiest way to put on the pounds is to eat your last meal of the day after 6:00 P.M. Most people are able to adhere to this schedule but it's impossible for me. I occasionally try to eat my largest meal at lunch but I thoroughly enjoy returning home from work in the evening and having a leisurely meal while watching my favorite TV shows. Consequently, I most often eat late and I don't have much of the evening left to burn off any of the calories that I consumed at dinner. I'm positive that if I could eat earlier in the evening each and every day, I would have no problem keeping my weight at a constant level.

Have you come to the obvious conclusion that this is a program of Behavior Modification? I'm sure you have. You don't need a degree in psychiatry, psychology, or social work to recognize it. It's merely COMMON SENSE. It isn't necessary to attend Amherst, Harvard, the University of West Virginia, or Yale. You don't even need to take any special mail order courses. You merely need to make up your mind that you're going to lose weight this time and that you're going to stick to the program.

The program embraces my daughter's doctrine — EAT LESS, EXERCISE MORE. The games you play, the crutches you choose, just take you to the next level. They give you the <u>tools</u> to work with to accomplish your weight loss goal.

LIVING LIFE —
THE REST OF THE STORY

By now you are completely aware that the name of this book is PLAYING GAMES – LOSING WEIGHT – LIVING LIFE.

I think I have sufficiently covered the various games in this program – the crutches that lead to eventual weight loss.

How many times have I used the phrases "you already know" or "I'm sure you know" while explaining this program? Definitely quite a few. That's because there certainly is no secret, and it really is perfectly obvious, which steps need to be taken to lose weight. Steps which you have heard or read about from every other diet program.

Now I'm going to explain why I added "Living Life" to the title of this book. I'm not going to try to tell you how to live <u>your</u> life, I'm just going to divulge some of the methods I use in my own to keep it running smoothly. I refer to them as "Hints For The Good Life".

I use the crutches, or the aids, or the tools, or however you want to refer to them, in many other phases of my life.

Basically, I'm a lazy person. I was born that way. I could very easily spend most of my day just being a couch potato. I do love to watch TV. I am addicted to "The Young and The Restless" and "The Bold and the Beautiful" to the point where I set my VCR when I need to be out at the time they air.

Because I recognized that fundamentally I <u>am</u> a lazybones, I knew I needed something to motivate me to accomplish what was necessary to be done.

First, I listed which household chores needed to be performed weekly. There was dusting, vacuuming, cleaning bathrooms, doing laundry, ironing and changing bed linens. I decided I would force myself to accomplish at least one of those tasks every day.

I then added two extra weekly duties of washing a window and doing an extra cleaning chore – one which only needs to be tackled monthly, or even only yearly. I was all set to put my plan into action.

The resolution was made with all the best of intentions but I still needed the motivation. I knew I didn't have the will power or the strength to do it on my own. For that reason I utilized my Christian upbringing and called upon my Lord to help me. I made a pledge to Him that every day I would accomplish one of the chores I had on my list.

Now when I do the particular job for the day I jot it down on my calendar. I use corresponding letters — D for dusting, V for vacuuming, C for cleaning bathrooms, L for laundry, I for ironing, B for changing the bed linens, E for an extra cleaning task, and W for cleaning a window. When you wash one window a week – you never need to tackle the entire house or apartment at one time or hire window cleaners.

See, I'm PLAYING THE GAME, accomplishing my tasks, getting a star and having fun. It may sound silly to you but it works for me. I'm amazed at how simple housework has become and how easy it is to keep my house clean.

When my daughter came upon my calendar one day she was quite concerned that the code meant I was keeping something about my health from her. When I told her what it was she nearly doubled over with laughter. She thinks I'm obsessive/compulsive. I never have confessed to her how lazy I really am. I guess she knows now.

I also play the game when there is an especially big project I want to undertake. For years I had just placed any snapshots I had taken into boxes. Sometimes I would date them and sometimes I wouldn't. I decided it was finally time to put my house in order and straighten out the snapshot mess. I vowed I would put them all in albums — and chronologically besides. I can never describe what a terribly humungous task it was! I had to use an entire room to spread out in.

For this tremendous task I promised to work at it for at least five minutes a day.

Most of the days I invested longer than the required five minutes, and before I knew it the project was completed. There were some days when I didn't have more than five minutes to spare (or I just didn't <u>feel </u>like working on it for more than the five minutes) but each day I always came five minutes closer to the completion.

Needless to say, when I take any snapshots now I almost always put them directly in the current album — or at least I date them on the back. I'll never go through that nightmare again.

I devised this program several years ago and I've been living it ever since. It has become a part of me. I can't imagine not playing the game. I don't need to choose a food crutch every day because I only need to <u>maintain</u> my weight loss— the weight I lost by using a different crutch every day. However, when I weigh myself each morning, if the scale tells me I have gained a pound, I'll choose a crutch and get back on the wagon.

HINTS FOR THE GOOD LIFE

I mentioned earlier that I would have a few hints for you. Most of them are household related but there is a hint for maintaining your health that has proved extremely helpful to me...

I obtained this information from a TV talk show. The topic was different kinds of home remedies for various health conditions.

Some were pretty far out, but then they brought up a remedy for arthritis.

My interest was peaked immediately because at that time of my life I had felt pain in both my thumbs and just knew it was the beginning of an arthritic condition. Some days it was worse than others – especially during inclement weather. There were several people in the audience who testified that they used the remedy and it either lessened or cured their arthritis.

I, and most of the audience, chuckled when we first heard what the remedy consisted of, but my interest was still peaked because of the unsolicited testimonials from the people in the audience. They swore that this remedy worked so I decided to give it a try. They weren't being compensated by a company. Now I'll give you the remedy. You'll probably chuckle yourself — or even laugh out loud — but I have to tell you, it <u>works.</u> Here it is:

Place a box of golden raisins (opened, of course) into a flat plastic or glass container and pour enough gin over them to cover. Yes, I said gin. Let them soak for approximately two weeks, or until they become saturated. Stir them occasionally. By the way, the dark raisins do not work.

When the raisins are thoroughly soaked you need to eat only nine of them per day. That's what the recipe recommended, however, I just take a teaspoonful before I retire in the evening. When the raisins get low I transfer them to a jar and start a new batch so I never run out.

Yes, I am still taking my raisin cure every night, and I started almost 12 years ago.

I rationalized that even if it didn't ease my pain, it couldn't hurt me. It was only food, after all, wasn't it? The pain in my thumbs subsided significantly after a few months and actually disappeared a couple of years after I started the regimen. If I have arthritis, I don't know it.

NEVER CLEAN YOUR SINKS AGAIN. Wipe your sinks and faucets with a dry towel each and every time you use them and you'll never have to scour again. They just won't get dirty and ugly water spots will be a thing of the past. Then too, if you have acidic water, the acidic deposits will not collect around the edges of the faucets causing that unsightly white calcification which is almost impossible to remove.

LOAD YOUR DISHWASHER by placing your forks in one area, the knives in another, and the spoons in another. You'll find it will be much faster to unload. Instead of having to pick out each one individually to return to your silverware drawer, you will be able to grab a bunch of each category in one CLEAN swoop. (Cool play on words, eh?)

IMMEDIATELY RETURN EACH ITEM TO ITS RIGHTFUL PLACE after you either prepare a meal, clean the house, try on different outfits, or whatever other activity you engage in. You probably do this anyway because it's only common sense, but it's surprising how many people don't. It's amazing how quickly things accumulate and clutter up a room. Using the same principle as "a stitch in time, saves nine", your entire house is constantly "picked up".

OPEN UP YOUR MAIL OVER THE RECYCLING BIN and the junk mail won't even have a chance to enter your house to clutter it up.

SCOTCH TAPE THE ENDS OF YOUR THREADS. My daughter thinks I'm out of my mind with this one, but I think it's cool. I keep seldom-used spools of colored thread in a box.

Finding the loose ends entangled together, I scotch-taped the end of the thread to the spool itself. Now, after I use the color I need, I just scotch tape it again. No more entangled ends, saving much time and aggravation. It's the little things in life that make it good!

FINAL WORDS

You have now learned all of my sage secrets of living the good life. You may give my program a shot or not, but in either case my book gave me the opportunity to inform you of just what options you have to change your life — if you so desire.

This attempt at writing is also a product of my program. Isn't it perfectly obvious that it's my first attempt? Believe me, I have a lot more respect for writers than I ever had before.

I promised my Lord that I would write at least one sentence a day, anticipating that I then would write at least a couple more. It worked. The words don't come easily to me and I'm absolutely positive that if I hadn't asked Him for help and made my promise to Him daily, I would have worked on it for a few days and then set it aside forever, never to be written.

I guess the old adage of learning how to walk before you can run applies here. You do it one step at a time. ONE DAY AT A TIME.

In this instance, it was one sentence at a time.

You now have forty-nine crutches to implement in order to lose the extra weight you have accumulated over the last few years. Those pounds which unmercifully sneaked up on you when you weren't constantly vigilant. It happens to all of us very easily.

Each day that you choose one of the crutches I suggested, (or one that you may think of yourself), and you put it into effect during the entire day, you <u>will</u> lose some calories. The amount you lose depends on the caloric count of the food you forsake for the day (or the efficiency of the particular discipline you chose to implement).

Once you've gotten hooked on the game, and I'm sure you will, you're going to have fun playing the "losing game" either by yourself, with your family, or wit(friends)Justhink— if each one of us would recruit one person to join the program, we could, feasibly, cure the American obesity disease. I am calling it a disease instead of just a problem because, in truth, it truly is a disease.

As I said in the beginning, there are so many "cures" for this disease— so many diets out there. Many of them don't produce any results at all, and those that do are very difficult to live with. They are usually abandoned after a short period of time.

PLAYING GAMES – LOSING WEIGHT – LIVING LIFE — is a program to which I can truthfully testify. I'm living proof that it <u>does work.</u> If you give it a chance it will work for you also.

Whenever our family discusses food (which is almost every time we get together), one of my grandsons always contributes a favorite, profound statement. It is:

"NO FOOD TASTES AS GOOD AS THE GOOD FEELING YOU GET FROM BEING THIN".

HE'S RIGHT, YOU KNOW.

Peg Grossi

ABOUT THE AUTHOR

The author is a seventy-eight-year old widow with two wonderful children, a son and a daughter, and four exceptional grandsons who help keep her young. She attributes her good health to the way of life described in her book. Her second love, after her family, is ballroom dancing. She tries to fit an evening into her busy schedule as often as possible. She studies tap dancing weekly and maintains it has helped to contribute to her excellent health. In addition, she loves to cook—and eat—which is what prompted her to write *PLAYING GAMES – LOSING WEIGHT – LIVING LIFE* to keep her weight under control.